Effortless Weight Loss

Your Keys to Unlocking Natural, Effortless Weight Loss & Maintenance

(Reversing & Managing Type 2 Diabetes & Obesity)

By Joseph C Fiorino, Jr DC

Dr Fiorino practices in Thayer, MO and can be reached at www.re-creatingyou.com

Special Thanks...

To my wife Sue chief editor, co-contributor, & still loves me when I'm buried in my projects. Without her I'd probably have lost my mind long ago.

Contents

Must Read!

It is the focus of my professional life to serve others not by merely directing them toward better health, but by helping them attain a higher quality of life. We were not meant to be miserable and drained of our joy to live. We were meant to express life more fully.

In the following pages, you'll read information that can...if you let it...change your life and for some of you, it could *save* your life. But, don't expect some magical solution, supplement, or pill. This isn't about fad diets; it's about eating what we were intended to eat the way we were intended to eat it.

The concepts are timeless and simple, but they are not necessarily easy. You will need to make some effort to reach your destination. So, you will need to decide *now* that you are ready and willing to do what it takes to get there. Please don't go into this with preconceived notions about what you thought was true. Set those aside and be ready to discard false information and replace it with what is true.

Are you ready? Then, let's get started on a new chapter...of better health and a better life.

Motivation

This is not a diet or some "gut it out for 8 weeks 'til I'm skinny" thing. This is ultimately about your health. Health is not a goal to be achieved or a destination that you get to then sit down and twiddle your thumbs.

Heath is on a continuum. At one end is life abundant and at the other end is death. You are either moving toward health or away from it and you'll only benefit from your healthy actions so long as you are doing them. Or, as I heard once, "Yesterday's homeruns don't win tomorrow's ballgames".

All of life is like this; there are no stops, no yields, no u-turns...you must keep going. So, don't fool yourself; you can't eat whatever you want, sit around doing nothing and expect to be lean and healthy.

On the positive side of things, you were made in the image of the Creator-God of the universe and you are worth the effort. Not, "it's" worth doing, or I'm doing this so I'll be better for my spouse, kids, etc...*You* have inherent value and you are worth it.

The Major Premise

We were intelligently designed by a Creator who established principles for how this body was intended to function right down to what fuel sources to use and for what. Even how those sources would interact with one another and organs inappropriately and the response to altered states of those fuels. Or, what nutrients were necessary for all of life's functions from growth and development to defending against foreign-microscopic invaders and damage to tissues and cells.

This body was made out of certain elements and for certain purposes. When those elements and purposes are altered, so is the body. Certainly we are living beings who can adapt and respond to our environments and not just a programmed system, but there is a "format" by which we are intended to run. Again, alter the format and you alter the ability for the being to adapt and respond the way it was intended...we get sick, fat, etc.

The Big "Fat" Lie

For a couple of decades we've been hearing that fat is the enemy and we're supposed to eat "lighter" to lose weight and be thin and healthy. But let's look at what eating fat free has done.

More than 2/3 of U.S Adults 20 & older are either overweight or obese. Half of that number or 1/3 of all adults 20 & older are obese. More than 12% of 2-5 years, 17% of 6-11, and 17% of 12-19 are overweight or obese. This costs an individual, on average, $1,429 *(42%)* more in health care costs. *(CDC statistics 2006)*

23.6 million *(7.8%)* children and adults in the U.S. have Type 2 Diabetes and 1.6 million new cases are diagnosed each year. *(Nat. Diabetes Fact Sheet 2007)*

81.1 million Americans have 1 or more forms of Cardiovascular Disease *(High blood pressure, coronary heart disease, stroke, heart failure)*. CVD is the leading cause of death in America. *(American Heart Assoc & CDC)*

We have been eating animal fats for eons *(what is now called saturated fat & blamed for CVD and weight gain)*. But, Cardiovascular "Diseases" on the other hand, have only been around since the 1940s or so which was right about the time when hydrogenated vegetable oils were introduced. Hmmmm.

You were made to use fat as both a fuel and a building material. In fact, it's our best fuel available; that's why we store it. The fats we consume are in the form of oils *(vegetable, canola)* or hydrogenated solids *(Margarine)* that our bodies can't use.

Yes, there are problems with some saturated fats, but not all of them are created equal. Feeding of grains to animals not made to consume them produce unhealthy fats rather than the incredibly healthy Omega-3 fatty acids they would produce if allowed to eat what they were designed to eat...grass.

Sugar's Deadly Secret

How can sugar be the problem? I know this sounds completely backwards, but read on to learn how our shift from traditional foods to processed foods is causing many of our health issues beyond just making us fatter.

Carbohydrates like breads, crackers, chips, processed food, refined flour..."sugars", are broken down to glucose. Glucose triggers the pancreas to produce insulin which sends the glucose into your cells be used for fuel.

Any glucose not used is stored in muscle and liver cells as glycogen for later use. Any glucose left in the bloodstream that isn't used and can't be stored gets converted to triglycerides in the liver and stored in fat cells or become sticky from insulin and clog your arteries.

High glucose from consuming too many carbs signals fat cells to not only store more fat/triglycerides, but also to hold on to fat and not release it for energy *(fat cells stay big)*. Eventually your muscle and liver cells become insulin resistant *(glycogen can't be stored)* and all excess carbs get stored as fat *(fat cells get bigger)*. Eventually diabetes results and, or heart disease.

Insulin is also very pro-inflammatory, creating pain in joints and muscles, and doing damage to those tissues. It causes your blood platelets to become sticky and causes the conversion of macrophages *(a white blood cell)* into foam cells *(they fill with cholesterol and build up in your arteries – "clogging of the arteries")*.

More Than Calories

Certainly there is a basic calorie in, calorie out scenario. If you eat more calories in a day than you can use, you will gain weight, but there's more to it than that.

Protein: Protein is for more than building muscle. Proteins and the amino acids that make them are the base components in making enzymes and hormones which are vital to life. Beyond this, they are also a high energy fuel source. You need approximately 0.5 – 1.0 grams of protein per pound of lean body mass per day, but your needs may be higher if your are either more physically active or a male.

Begin to move proteins out of the weight room and into body fuel category. It's not our primary source of energy, but it is much more useful than is typically recognized.

Fats: Fats are our primary and longest lasting fuel for our body. It is also critical in building healthy cells of all kinds in our body. All cell walls are made of fats *(lipids)* and cholesterols. Also, cholesterols are used to build many of our hormones.

Conventional wisdom has said that eating fat makes us fat, but this is absolutely wrong.

When we have excess fat in our diets and there is no insulin in the blood stream, the body will respond by raising the metabolic rate *(increased cell activity to burn more calories, even at rest)* and by increasing the production of ketones *(another useful fuel source)*.

However, not all fats are created equal. Fats can be divided between man-made fats *(processed foods, partially hydrogenated vegetable oils, and grain fed animal products)* and God-made fats *(meats, eggs, dairy, fish, nuts, seeds, omega-3 oils)*. So, yes, eating man-made fats do contribute to the storing of fats simply because your body doesn't know what to do with it.

Carbohydrates: Carbs are used only as a fuel source. They serve no other function in the body. *Carbohydrates control insulin & insulin controls fat storage.* There are simple and complex carbs, but both eventually become glucose. I want you to begin to think: carbohydrates = sugar; even those brown breads at the store that claim to be "whole grain".

With carbohydrates as the primary food source spikes in insulin not only result in heart & vascular problems, but unstable energy levels, mood swings, and decreased libido. If carbs = sugar, then it also suppresses your immune system by at least 20% for up to 5 hours after eating it.   They also trigger the inflammatory cascade which leads to general pain and stiffness.

You may have even noticed that when you eat that bagel at 7am you're hungry again by 9:30 or 10.   There are plenty of calories to keep you going that long, but these simple carbs keep triggering the insulin response that tells your brain it needs more energy even when you haven't used that energy...So, you go grab another snack/carb and the vicious cycle keeps going.

Good carbs versus bad carbs.   Bad carbs are simple "sugars" *(breads, pastas, crackers, pretzels, cookies, cakes, sweets, pastries, bagels, breakfast cereals, white rice, sodas, sweet drinks, all processed foods – made from refined flower devoid of any real nutritional value – like biscuits, pancakes, waffles).*

Here are a couple of examples: A large soda (32oz) has 98 grams of sugar.   That's almost ½ a cup of sugar in 1 drink! Would you even dream of scooping up a ½ cup of sugar just to eat?   A 2-liter has 216 grams (7.71oz) or almost a full cup of sugar.   A ¾ cup serving of pasta has 41 grams (1.46oz) of carbs/sugar. That's almost a fifth of a cup of sugar.

Read those labels: Let's take a "healthy" Nutri-Grain® bar. On the ingredients list are enriched flower *(enriched because they had to add back in only a handful of the nutrients stripped out and replaced with synthetic sources)*, high fructose corn syrup, sugar, calcium carbonate *(cancer causing)*, whey, wheat gluten, corn starch...that's not even the filling. All of these contribute to triggering the effects of glucose discussed previously.

Good carbs are nutrient dense like vegetables and fruits *(there are 2 extensive lists later...keep reading)*.

Ask yourself this question. Where were all of those processed foods in the beginning? The farther we get away from the way our foods were either growing out of the ground or moving around on this earth, the less beneficial and potentially harmful it is to us.

Back to the Major Premise: **This body was made out of certain elements and for certain purposes. When those elements and purposes are altered, so is the body.**

Make It Effortless

Your goal to get the scale moving in the right direction is essentially to get the processed carbs and sugars out of your life. Do that, and you'll begin to not only effortlessly lose weight, but keep it off as well. I'm going to give you 3 general categories though in order to get your bearings. Weight Loss, Maintenance, and Weight Gain.

Weight Loss:

Anything under 100 grams of carbohydrates per day will result in effortless weight loss. The lower you go, the quicker and easier the weight will come off. Anything 40 grams or less will result in more significant losses. This can be done 1 to 2 days at a time for more aggressive weight loss.

Don't stay here too long if you're just trying to shed a few pounds or you will deplete your glycogen stores and begin to feel fatigued and gittery. Not to mention that you're limiting intake of vital nutrients from fruits and veggies. *(Eat all the green, red, & yellow veg you want – except corn)*

* For the Obese and/or Type 2 Diabetics. You can extend your stay in this range *(Please be*

supervised by a healthcare provider). Some of you will need to be under 10 grams per day to be in this range. Again, don't stay here too long *(not more than 5-6 days at a time)*...you will be eliminating your nutrient rich fruits and veggies and should be taking a multi-vitamin supplement.

Stay in this range until you reach your best weight. Remember, this is about your health and not getting skinny. Once you get to a weight that fits your build and energy level requirements move into the following range to maintain this healthy weight...for life.

Maintenance:

Staying just over the 100 gram *(3.52 oz)* mark with your primary intake of carbohydrates coming from vegetables and fruits and minimal intake of the right kinds of grains *(see the list starting on p25)* will result in effortless weight maintenance. You'll be eating well and staying surprisingly satisfied between meals eating in this range.

As you make this "home" and a part of your lifestyle, you'll experience more consistent energy and less of an appetite. You'll also be consistently reversing the effects of diabetes and other cardiovascular problems. Jump too far

18

above this and you'll be back in the yo-yo syndrome of energy drops and cravings.

Weight Gain:

Somewhere over 150 grams *(5.29 oz)* of carbs per day is insidious weight gain and a very unhealthy, shortened life. Amazingly, the U.S. Department of Health & Human Services recommends from 170-226 grams *(6-8 oz)* of simple, poor carbohydrates per day in addition to fruits and vegetables *(2010 Dietary Guidelines – Food Pyramid)*. Is it any wonder we're having so many health issues in this country?

As you can imagine, many Americans are well over the 150g amount. Here's an example: 3 pancakes *(no syrup)* – 63g, 1 bagel *(snack at break)* – 45g, plate of spaghetti for lunch – 81g, a couple of slices of pizza for dinner – 80g, 2lg sodas *(lunch & dinner)* – 196g, and a slice of cake for dessert *(because you deserve it)* – 33g...for a grand total of 498g of carbs/sugar. Cut it in half and you are still at 249g.

* Don't let some of those thin people eating bad carbs fool you. They are only moderating calories. Underneath, they are still producing the same terrible effects we've already discussed. Remember, the goal is healthy, not just thin.

What Then Shall We Eat?

What we eat is critical. It is the vast majority of what determines whether we will lose or gain weight. Other factors include physical activity and other healthy lifestyle habits.

A very small percentage is related to genetics. The field of epigenetics has shown us that we can actually switch genes on and off. Change your life and you can actually change your genes *(you'll need to change your jeans too before long)*.

Unfortunately, the most widely known pattern is the Food Pyramid. Even the updated one and the diabetic food pyramid are skewed in the wrong direction. Your primary intake of food should consist of...

First: Vegetables & Fruits *(Refer to the previous chapter for amount of carbs)* – This will represent the majority of your meal and nutrients.

Second: Meat, Fish, Fowl, Eggs, and Dairy – This will be your major source of calories *(Because these are slow burners, you will feel satisfied longer between meals while maintaining your energy)*.

Third: Nuts & Seeds – Keep these handy for snacks or for extra flavors and texture with other foods.

Fourth: Herbs, Spices, Extracts – Season your food all you want. They have other health benefits as well.

Fifth: Grains – Keep these to a minimum. Some of them, like quinoa are more protein than carb and are loaded with other nutrients. If you grind your own wheat berries *(like my wife does...goddess)* you can keep some bread in the mix.

To keep it simple you need to become what I call a "Perimeter Shopper". Stay to the perimeter, or the outer boundaries of the grocery store. That's where all of the *real* food is; the meats, eggs, dairy, fish, fruits, and vegetables are. The inner aisles have primarily processed foods that are not only contributing to weight gain, but are also loaded with chemicals and other toxins that are harmful to us. In other words, if it's in a box, bag, or can, its probably bad for you.

CAUTION 1: When cooking, go back to using butter, ghee or olive oil. I know this is contrary to the "wisdom" of the day...In short; these are fats your body recognizes as usable *(God-made)* and studies show they are not what are clogging our arteries. Vegetable, Canola, etc. types of oils are unstable, become rancid and cancer causing with heat. Your best way to cook is to steam. The vast majority of your fruits and vegetables can be eaten raw.

CAUTION 2: Dried fruit is an excellent option, but be sure to read the label. Many are prepared with either sugar or high fructose corn syrup. And in general are higher in sugar, snack on these in moderation. The same goes for trail mixes. Watch out for processed, high sugar yogurt-covered raisins, M&M's and other candies.

Set Yourself Up For Success

1. Discipline: If it's going to happen, it's up to you. You are the only one who can do it. So, tell your inner brat to sit down and be quiet so you can accomplish this and make it permanent. Ask yourself how bad you want to lose the weight and be healthier and decide today that your indulgences aren't worth it.

2. Go Team: Find yourself at least one person who will support you in this process. Call for encouragement or to share your successes. Even if you have to go outside your own home, it's worth it.

3. Clean House: Get all of the processed carbs and sweets out of your house. The temptation will be too strong, especially in the heat of the moment. You're not depriving yourself of anything, if those foods are stealing your health and slowly killing you.

4. Stock Up: Make sure you have plenty of acceptable foods available *(refer to the lists below).* If it's not there, you shouldn't eat it... and stopping by your favorite fast food restaurant or just ordering a pizza won't work. *(Yes, pizza is made with refined/processed flour and is just sugar)*

Stock up on what? On the following pages are a couple of lists. One is a list of some of the healthiest foods you can possibly eat and the reason why they are so beneficial. The second is a list of other exceptionally wonderful foods. So, just take your pick and keep the fridge and pantry full of these wonderful foods.

The Healthiest Foods Ever Made

This is a list of foods which will be the most nutrient dense to get more out of the carb calories you'll be consuming, as well as decrease your risk for deadly illnesses like cancer, diabetes and heart disease. To calculate for your best place on the carb curve for effortless weight loss take the percentage of sugar per gram weight from the total grams of a given food. *(100g blueberries x 0.10 [10%] = 10g of sugar, figure approximately 2% for all vegetables – 1oz = 28g)*

Fruits

Blueberries
Antioxidants, which prevents free-radical damage *(pre-cancer cells)* and supports the immune system and protects the heart. One serving can provide 30% of your RDA of vitamin C. 10% sugar per gram weight. Keep them fresh or frozen *(let thaw for a few minutes)* and munch down a handful a day, just for the health of it.

Apricots
Beta-carotene, which helps prevent free-radical damage and protect the eyes. The body also turns beta-carotene into vitamin A, which may help ward off some cancers, especially of the skin. 10% sugar per gram weight. Snack

on them dried, or if you prefer fresh, buy when still firm; once they soften, they lose nutrients.

Avocados
Oleic acid, an unsaturated fat that helps lower overall cholesterol and raise levels of HDL, plus a good dose of fiber. 1% sugar per gram weight. Try a few slices instead of mayonnaise to dress up your next burger.

Raspberries
Ellagic acid, which helps stall cancer-cell growth and loaded with antioxidants. These berries are also packed with vitamin C and are high in fiber, which helps prevent high cholesterol and heart disease. 6% sugar per gram weight. Top plain low-fat yogurt or oatmeal (another high fiber food) with fresh berries. *(Very similar in nature to the newly popular Acai berries)*

Mango
A medium mango packs 57mg of vitamin C, almost your whole-recommended daily dose. This antioxidant helps prevent arthritis and boosts wound healing and your immune system. Mangoes also boast more than 8,000 IU of vitamin A *(as beta-carotene)*. 16% sugar per gram weight.

Cantaloupe

Vitamin C *(117mg in half a melon, almost twice the recommended daily dose)* and beta-carotene – both powerful antioxidants that help protect cells from free-radical damage. Plus, half a melon has 853mg of potassium – almost twice as much as a banana, which helps lower blood pressure. 8% sugar per gram weight. Cut into cubes and freeze, then blend into an icy smoothie.

Cranberries & Juice

Helps fight bladder infections by preventing harmful bacteria from growing. 6% sugar per gram weight. Buy 100 percent juice concentrate and use it to spice up your daily water without adding sugar. Look out for added sugar in the juices.

Tomato

Lycopene, one of the strongest carotenoids, acts as an antioxidant. Research shows that tomatoes may cut the risk of bladder, stomach and colon cancers in half if eaten daily. 3% sugar per gram weight. Drizzle fresh slices with olive oil, because lycopene is best absorbed when eaten with a little fat.

Raisins

These little gems are a great source of iron, which helps the blood transport oxygen and which many women are short on. 60% sugar per gram weight – so be careful. Sprinkle raisins on your morning oatmeal or bran cereal – women, consider this especially during your period.

Figs
A good source of potassium and fiber, figs also contain vitamin B6, which is responsible for producing mood-boosting serotonin, lowering cholesterol and preventing water retention. 50% sugar per gram weight – so be careful. Fresh figs are delicious simmered alongside a pork tenderloin and the dried variety make a great portable snack.

Lemons/Limes
Limonene, furocoumarins and vitamin C, all of which help prevent cancer. 2% sugar per gram weight. Buy a few of each and squeeze over salads, fish, beans and vegetables for fat free flavor.

Vegetables

Onions
Quercetin is one of the most powerful flavonoids (*natural plant antioxidants*). Studies show it helps protect against cancer. Chop onions for the maximum phytonutrient boost, or if you hate to cry, roast them with a little butter or olive oil and serve with rice or other vegetables.

Artichokes

These odd-looking vegetables contain silymarin, an antioxidant that helps prevent skin cancer, plus fiber to help control cholesterol. Steam over boiling water for 30 to 40 minutes. Squeeze lemon juice on top, then pluck the leaves off with your fingers and use your teeth to scrape off the rich-tasting skin. When you get to the heart, you have found the best part!

Ginger

Gingerols may help reduce queasiness; other compounds may help ward off migraines and arthritis pain by blocking inflammation-causing prostaglandins. Peel the tough brown skin and slice or grate into a stir-fry.

Broccoli

Indole-3-carbinol and sulforaphane, which help protect against breast and other cancers. Broccoli also has lots of vitamin C and beta-carotene. Don't overcook broccoli – instead, steam lightly to preserve phytonutrients. Squeeze fresh lemon on top for a zesty and taste, added nutrients and some vitamin C.

Spinach

Lutein and zeaxanthin, carotenoids that help fend off macular degeneration, a major cause of blindness in older people. Plus, studies show this green fountain of youth may help to reverse some signs of aging. Add raw leaves to a salad or sautéed with a little butter/olive oil and garlic.

Bok Choy *(Chinese cabbage)*
Brassinin, which some research suggests may help prevent breast tumors, plus indoles and isothiocyanates, which lower levels of estrogen, make this vegetable a double-barreled weapon against breast cancer. A cup will also give you 158mg of calcium *(16 percent of your daily recommended requirement)* to help beat osteoporosis. Find it in your grocer's produce section or an Asian market. Slice the greens and juicy white stalks, then sauté like spinach or toss into a stir-fry just before serving.

Squash *(Butternut, Pumpkin, Acorn...)*
Winter squash has huge amounts of vitamin C and beta-carotene, which may help protect against endometrial cancer. Cut one in half, scoop out the seeds and bake with a Tbs of butter in scooped out portion until soft, then dust with cinnamon.

Watercress and Arugula
Phenethyl isothiocyanate, which, along with beta-carotene and vitamins C and E, may help keep cancer cells at bay. Do not cook these leafy greens; instead, use them to garnish a sandwich or add a pungent, peppery taste to a salad.

Garlic

The sulfur compounds that give garlic its pungent flavor can also lower LDL "bad" cholesterol, lower blood pressure and even reduce your risk of stomach and colon cancer, and is a natural anti-biotic/viral *(juice a clove & fill the rest of the glass with carrot juice for colds)*. Bake a whole head for 15 to 20 minutes, until soft and sweet and spread on bread instead of butter.

Grains, Beans and Nuts

Quinoa *(Pronounced Keen-Wah)*

A half cup of cooked quinoa has 5 grams of protein, more than any other grain, plus iron, riboflavin and magnesium. Add to soup for a protein boost. Rinse first, or it will taste bitter.

Wheat Germ

A tablespoon gives you about 7 percent of your daily magnesium, which helps prevent muscle cramps; it is also a good source of vitamin E. Sprinkle some over yogurt, fruit or cereal.

Lentils

Isoflavones, which may inhibit estrogen-promoted breast cancers, plus fiber for heart health and an impressive 9 grams of protein per half cup. Isoflavones hod up through processing, so buy lentils dried or already in a soup. Take them to work, and you will have a protein packed lunch.

Peanuts

Studies show that peanuts or other nuts *(which contain mostly unsaturated "good" fat)* can lower your heart-disease risk by over 20 percent. Recent studies show peanuts to be very high in antioxidants. Keep a packet in your briefcase, gym bag or purse for a protein-packed post-workout boost or an afternoon pick me up that will satisfy you until supper, or chop a few into a stir-fry for a Thai accent.

Pinto Beans

A half cup has more than 25 percent of your daily requirement of folate, which helps protect against heart disease and reduces the risk of birth defects. Great in a pot of vegetarian chili.

Yogurt

Beneficial bacteria in active-culture yogurt helps prevent yeast infections; calcium strengthens bones. Get the plain kind and mix in your own fruit to keep calories and sugar down. If you are lactose intolerant, never fear – yogurt should not bother your tummy.

Dairy, Eggs and Seafood

Raw Milk

Riboflavin *(a.k.a. vitamin B2)* is important for good vision and along with vitamin A might help improve eczema and allergies. Plus, you get calcium and vitamin D, too.

Eggs *(Free-range organic)*
They have all of the 22 amino acids, 2g sugar, and if they are allowed to eat grass and bugs they create quite a bit of Omega-3 fatty acids. Except for vitamin C, they have all other vitamins including the B vitamins *(especially B_{12} & Riboflavin)*, and one of the few food sources of vitamin D. They are loaded with minerals like iodine, phosphorous & potassium...and best of all you can raise them in your own backyard.

Shellfish *(Clams, Mussels)*
Vitamin B12 to support nerve and brain function, plus iron and hard-to-get minerals like magnesium and potassium. Try a bowl of tomato-based Manhattan clam chowder.

Salmon
Cold-water fish like salmon, mackerel and tuna are the best sources of omega-3 fatty acids, which help reduce the risk of cardiac disease. Brush fillets with ginger-soy marinade and broil until fish flakes easily with a fork.

Crab
A great source of vitamin B12 and immunity-boosting zinc. The "crab" in sushi is usually made from fish; buy it fresh or pre-cooked instead and make your own crab cakes.

Your Expanded Foods List
Take Your Pick & Enjoy!

Vegetables:

Asparagus	Avocados
Beets *	Bell peppers
Broccoli	Brussels sprouts
Cabbage	Carrots *
Cauliflower	Celery
Collard Greens	Cucumbers
Eggplants	Fennel
Garlic	Green beans
Green peas	Kale
Leeks	Mushrooms
Mustard greens	Olives
Onions	Potatoes *
Romaine lettuce	Spinach
Squash	Sweet potatoes
Swiss chard	Tomatoes
Turnip greens	Zucchini

Fruits:

Apples *	Apricots
Bananas *	Blackberries
Blueberries	Cantaloupe
Cranberries	Figs *
Grapefruit	Grapes *
Kiwifruit	Lemon/Lime
Oranges	Papaya

Pears	Pineapple
Plums	Prunes
Raisins *	Raspberries
Strawberries	Watermelon

Poultry & Lean Meat:

Beef, grass fed	Chicken
Lamb	Turkey
Venison/Deer	Rabbit

Fish & Seafood:

Bass	Catfish
Cod	Crappie
Flounder	Halibut
Salmon	Sardines
Scallops	Shrimp
Swordfish	Trout
Tuna	

Eggs & Dairy:

Cheese	Eggs
Kefir	Milk, cow/goat
Yogurt	

Nuts & Seeds:

Almonds	Cashews
Flaxseeds	Peanuts
Pecans	Pumpkin seeds
Sesame seeds	Sunflower seeds
Walnuts	

Beans & Legumes:

Black beans

Lentils

Pinto beans *

Tempeh *

Kidney beans

Lima beans *

Soybeans

Tofu *

Grains:

Barley

Buckwheat

Oats

Rye

Brown rice

Millet

Quinoa

Wheat *(if ground at home & used sparingly)*

Spices & Herbs:

Basil

Chili pepper

Coriander seeds

Cloves

Dill

Oregano

Peppermint

Sage

Turmeric

Cayenne pepper

Cilantro

Cinnamon

Cumin

Mustard seeds

Parsley

Rosemary

Thyme

Natural Sweeteners:

(Use sparingly)

Blackstrap molasses

Honey

Stevia

Cane juice

Maple syrup

CAUTION 1: Anything with an asterisk (*) after it are higher in sugar – stay away from these during weight loss periods and focus on the green, red, & yellow veggies 1st then fruits 2nd.

CAUTION 2: Many people have wheat/gluten sensitivities or to other grains and can hinder your progress. This could be a sign of an overgrowth of yeast in your gut. Many experience bloating and other digestive problems, or migraines. Please contact Dr. Fiorino if you experience any of these problems for help. Simple lab work can be done to test.

Buy Organic: If you're going to make the most of it, it pays to buy organic. Why? Because of toxins/chemicals in and on the foods. The large scale, mono-culture *"pharming"* practices used require chemical fertilizers, chemical pesticides and herbicides, or they've genetically modified the true identity out of the food. If your liver and other detoxing organs can't keep up with the load to get it out of your body, the liver will at least wrap a toxin/chemical in fat and, you guessed it...store it away to protect your body from its harmful effects.

Cooking: For more traditional methods of preparing and cooking foods the way our bodies were intended to consume these delicious foods refer to *Nourishing Traditions,* by Sally Fallon.

Frozen foods are acceptable, but you really should stay away from canned because of the chemical preservatives and the foods can pick up some of the aluminum *(especially if they are dented – aluminum leads to Alzheimer's).* If you do get canned, read those labels. The cheaper brands usually don't waste money on preservatives.

Watch out for the condiments. Again, read the labels and go for the cheaper brands. Heinz Ketchup is made from concentrate and has high fructose corn syrup, regular corn syrup and other seasonings. A cheaper brand we use has tomatoes and salt. Big difference. If you use peanut butter, look for the natural or organic. Jif®, for example, adds molasses, hydrogenated vegetable oil (rapeseed & soybean) and mono- & diglycerides. Smucker's Natural just has peanuts and less than 1% of salt.

Small Scale Do-it-Yourself
And other natural things

With a little effort, you can plant your own garden and get quality foods, some work/exercise, and some sunshine to make vit. D. You'll even save a little money on your grocery budget.

A few chickens in your backyard *(you'd be surprised where you're allowed to keep them)* will keep you supplied with some incredibly nutrient rich eggs for omelets, quiche, etc.

You could even raise your own meats. Chicken and rabbit are the easiest and require very little space. You can raise them right in your back yard. Rabbit is quite possibly the healthiest meat there is. If you live in a rural area you could raise beef, but be sure to stick with grass only for the healthiest animal and product.

Rural areas also have a wide range of edibles in the wild. There's deer, turkey, squirrel, rabbit, etc. Not to mention blackberries, mulberries, and mushrooms *(careful!)*. Don't forget walnuts, pecans, and other nuts. So many wonderful options that are delicious and good for you.

Making It Practical & Simple

If doing the math is overwhelming, focus primarily on eating until you feel *satisfied* and not *full*. Being more accurate can help with those "last few pounds". Slow down, chew and enjoy your food; it takes a while for your brain to catch up with your stomach. Remember, the primary issue is carbs/sugars. If you're going to watch something more closely, put your efforts there.

I do want you to be prepared for a pitfall. The rest of the world isn't really set up to consume food this way. So, when you go out to eat or to someone else's home for dinner...what do you do? They may think you're crazy, but trust me, it's worth it. Say no to the pasta salad, but eat the veggies in it or get the cottage cheese instead. Say no to the bun, but eat the burger.

Did you really look at that list of foods? That's a lot of wonderful food. What I've presented to you in this booklet is how we were made to eat. We have been given some rather tasty, God-made foods that are there to richly nourish us, not just to sustain life, but to have vibrant life abundantly.

Beyond food, the two most significant things you can do to improve your health and support your weight loss are...

1. Drink plenty of water. You should be drinking at least ¼ of your body weight in ounces. If you weigh 160 pounds, then you need to be drinking a minimum of 40oz of water per day. This is critical to support all of the metabolic activity your body is doing. Also, water keeps you from drinking sugar and calories that you need to be eating.

2. Get plenty of rest. 7-9 hours of sleep is ideal. This relates to your adrenal glands *(they secrete cortisol in response to increases in blood sugar and insulin).* If they are constantly at work dealing with carbs/sugar, they need a chance to shut off. If you don't get enough sleep, you further fatigue those adrenals and that leads to overall fatigue. If you are one to get that second wind and just stay up late, plan to get to bed before that and you'll start to wake up refreshed more often and take the weight off more easily.

Exercise Principles

I hesitate to even say "exercise", because it evokes images of trips to the gym, aerobics classes, weight rooms...or a trainer screaming at you to do two more. The only real reason we exercise is because we don't work and do the physical activity we used to...We're Lazy. By making everything convenient and inventing technology that does everything for us, we've contributed to our own diminishing health. We drive everywhere instead of walking. We buy our food instead of planting and harvesting it. We sit at desks instead of doing physical labor.

That being said, it's really about moving your body enough day to day to burn the calories that you eat. So, be creative with the following principles. *(Also, refer to the Special Note for Seniors...it's not just for seniors)*

1. Keep Moving: Walk, hike, bike, swim...do something at an easy to moderate rate 3-6 hours a week. *(This is not running/jogging)* It could be simple things like parking a little farther away, walking to the end of your ¼ mile lane instead of driving to get the mail; you get the idea.

2. Work Those Muscles: To burn up those stores of glycogen in muscles other than our legs from walking, to stimulate greater metabolic activity, and to just use it or lose it you need to use some other muscles. This could be by using light to heavy weights for brief but fairly intense full body exercises. They should be highly functional movements *(movements you would actually do in real life)*, so this could be doing chores if you have a garden or animals, yard work *(mowing the lawn)*, cleaning the house and doing laundry.

3. Go All Out: About once a week or so you should do something that really gets your heart pumping whether it be jogging, playing basketball or tennis, cutting wood...etc. It should be fairly intense *(you'll probably break a sweat and breath heavy)*. If you can get in even just 10 minutes once a week, it will stimulate further needs to burn any stored glycogen in your muscles and liver as well as fat cells.

Even walking 20-30 minutes a day for 5 out of 7 days in a week will make a huge difference. Physical activity has **three major benefits**...1. Burning of any extra calories that might otherwise be stored. 2. Increasing your body's rate of metabolism *(general cellular activity)*. 3. "Training" your body to not store fat *(it becomes more ready to use it for the physical activity)*

Bottom line, use your body and keep moving. We were made to move and work. Get out and enjoy this beautiful creation, breath deep and spend time doing something with those you love. You'll be happier, healthier and oh yeah, you'll lose some weight.

A Special Note For Seniors

From birth until somewhere into our 30's the average person is constantly rebuilding all of there body's cells, tissues, and organs. The rate of new cells replacing old cells is faster as we are growing. But, once we've stopped growing it slows to just a maintenance rate throughout the majority of our life.

When we begin to hit our 50's or so the rate of cells dying to the rate of cells regenerating is faster. This means two things... 1. You gain weight easier & 2. You are slowly deteriorating.

However, the greater requirement we put on our bodies to rebuild, the better we can keep up with the cell death rate. In plain English, physical activity that is enough to fatigue and break down muscle, make your heart pump more blood, lungs exchange more oxygen...etc. will require that your body rebuild it, use it, keep all cell activity *(metabolism)* up. Your body recognizes that it still needs to keep up with these demands and does. So, the younger you can get active and stay active, the better.

Final Note

If, for some reason you find yourself struggling to lose the weight, there may be some simple reasons why. It could be that other aspects of your health are hindering progress. It is common for people to have dysbiosis *(an imbalance between the good & bad bacteria in your gut)* or issues with a sluggish thyroid and/or adrenal fatigue; some have food allergies that can hinder them...These and others can contribute to difficulty losing weight and improving your health. You are welcome to consult the doctor to discuss & analyze your situation.

I wish you well on your journey and I have hope for your success. If you'll believe in yourself that you can do it, you'll get there. Remember, everything in life is a process and the vast majority of things worth having or doing are not about instant gratification. Be patient, stick with the plan and you'll do great.

God Bless,

Joe Fiorino, DC

If you have been helped by the information found in this booklet, please let others know. Send them to www.re-creatingyou.com. You can contact Dr Fiorino here as well.

About The Author

Dr. Fiorino maintains a Chiropractic practice in the beautiful Ozarks of Southern Missouri. He specializes as a Wellness Chiropractor seeing patients with health issues ranging from cancers, seizures, multiple digestive problems, chronic illnesses, heart and respiratory illnesses, urinary incontinence, asthmas & allergies...and many other health problems.

He emphasizes restoring the whole person back to the way they were created and not the treatment of symptoms. Look for his book *Re-Creating You* to continue your journey of restoring and maintaining your best health possible.